TRANSFORMATION
IT'S ONLY BRAIN SURGERY

Ann Lisette Wesso

ISBN: 1475043376
ISBN 13: 9781475043372

ODE: Intimations of Immortality

Our birth is but a sleep and a forgetting
The soul that rises with us, our life's Star,
Hath had elsewhere its setting,
And cometh from afar:
Not in entire forgetfulness,
And not in utter nakedness,
But trailing clouds of glory do we come
From God, who is our home.

William Wordsworth

CHAPTERS

DEDICATION

This book is dedicated to my family and dear friends who prayed and loved me during this experience. I could literally feel your love and kindness. If anyone is to be thanked even more it would be my brother, Bill Wesso, who returned from Florida to be with me for which I am truly grateful.

DISCLAIMER

This is not a testimonial to any one form of healing. It is simply my account of all the experiences that happened to me. I respectfully retell the facts as I interpret them. It is meant to be a guide for others to consider, and not a reflection of condemnation for those who have more serious conditions. The procedures and techniques are not meant to substitute for the medical advice of a professional. Please consult your medical professional before adopting any of the suggestions in this book. If someone is unwilling to accept responsibility for their own choices, I suggest they don't read this. The author and publisher disclaim any liability arising directly or indirectly from the use of this book.

ACKNOWLEDGMENTS

First of all, I want to thank God for giving me the talent and focus to express myself in writing this book and who allowed me to recover completely in such a short time from this very intense experience.

I would like to acknowledge and thank several people who helped me through my surgery. Firstly, to my brother, Bill Wesso, for completely supporting me through this experience, and his wife, Connie, for being so gracious and kind; to Lewie Wesso, my nephew, who stayed at the hospital the entire day of my surgery and actually drove me to buy a recliner the day before so I could recover in comfort.

I would also like to acknowledge Pat Pollock who drove me to and from the hospital and all of my doctor appointments and has been a true friend; to Lewie Pollock for taking my picture that appears on the back of this book; to Kathy Guy, the choir director, who led prayers for me and drove me to church several times; to all of St. Joseph's Choir who prayed for me and who are like a family; and to Doug Goertzen, who visited me in the hospital. In addition, thanks to all those who sent cards and flowers. For all these people I am truly grateful.

INTRODUCTION

This is a true story. It is a story about me and my brain tumor. It is a blend between the scientific, allopathic side of medicine and the natural, alternative side of medicine. Overall, including recent developed techniques, they provide the best care medicine has to offer at the current time.

I've been extremely blessed to experience these techniques and benefit from them. Obviously, things will change in the future as new technology is discovered. In addition, we must remember to integrate the "ancient" ways of the mystics and shamans so they are not lost or forgotten, so that our souls may thrive.

In my opinion, this is a combination of the most advanced aspects of modern medicine plus techniques from ancient times that work toward complete physical and emotional wholeness. These are modern miracles.

> *"Sometimes to see the light, we must bend it through the prism of illness."*

Julian Kalmar, Founder, 10 Million Clicks for Peace

CHAPTER 1

THE BEGINNING...

People simply do not understand brain surgery or brain tumors. I know, because I didn't understand it either! In fact, when I mention this to others, they are very shocked. This is the reason I am writing this book.

My diagnosis was a shock for me to say the least. People often say, "It's not exactly brain surgery," to describe something easy, yet, in this case, it was brain surgery, and it was mine.

Two years ago I experienced my first seizure. I was living in Reno. I did not understand what happened because I couldn't quite grasp it. When I thought about it later, I never in a million years expected the diagnosis.

This is the beginning of my incredible journey. It was a transformation of my body, mind and soul. Though I've had many interesting and profound experiences throughout my life, this one is symbolic of a rebirth to my being; a change in attitude and perception of life itself.

*"We don't see things as they are,
we see things as we are."*

Anais Nin

CHAPTER 2

MY FIRST SEIZURE

My eyes and arms grasped towards the ceiling. Unformed words attempted to come out of my mouth that I couldn't quite articulate. What was happening? Suddenly, I panicked and passed out... all in a split second.

I regained consciousness and found myself face down on the floor. As I slowly came back to consciousness, I pulled myself up and went into the bathroom to clean myself. Then, I called Nina, a friend who lived down the hall. I asked her to come and help me, and she showed up in seconds. She said I was quite pale, but who wouldn't be after passing out for forty-five minutes. I know it was this amount of time because I burned a pan of food on the stove. Nina was more worried than I. For some reason, I didn't react the same way as she did.

Prior to this episode, I had considered moving back to Pekin, Illinois. Pekin was where I was raised until fourth grade. At the time, I was living in Reno and wasn't very happy. I had just split up with my boyfriend of over one year, or rather he split up with me. Then within a month, he married. I had a difficult time making sense of all this because he kept telling me his relationship with the other woman was strictly business. Foolish me, I believed him. It was, no doubt, "monkey business." How naïve could I be? Obviously, this is a sign of some unfinished business within myself.

However, in that particular moment, I knew what I had to do. I had to move back to Pekin. No question in my mind or heart.

I called my brother, Bill, and asked if it would be possible for me to move back to Pekin and if I could stay with him for a couple weeks. I then told him about my seizure; he was very concerned. Initially, he wanted to fly to Reno to help me drive back. However, realizing he would not fit into my little car (I have a Saturn and he's over six feet tall), he let me drive on my own. Not sure about the wisdom in that choice, yet I was okay about it. Even though I was dubious of the trip, I managed it rather well, if I do say so myself.

In the end, I followed my intuition and am glad **because I believe my neurosurgery is the entire reason I moved to Illinois.**

"As human beings, our greatness lies not so much in being able to remake the world…as in being able to remake ourselves."

Mahatma Ghandi

CHAPTER 3

MY DRIVE BACK TO ILLINOIS

I left Reno at the beginning of October, 2009, and made the long trip back to Pekin in five days. Somehow, I didn't expect it to be such a long and exhausting drive. Not surprisingly, I was very tired at the end of each day and at the end of the trip.

I spent the night in several motels along the way. Some were better than others. I especially remember the last one because it was in the middle of a cornfield. It was a brand new motel. The manager was nice and very helpful especially when I complained about too much light coming in through the windows. I like it pitch black when I sleep, so the manager and I stuffed towels around the windows to keep out the light. In the morning, I was anxious to get going because it was my last day on the road and only had about 250 miles to drive. I had driven to exhaustion the day before. So, I got up extra early, ate a continental breakfast, checked out, and was on my merry way.

It was raining when I arrived in East Peoria. I met my brother, Bill, at a local restaurant. My brother's friend Dick was there and asked me, "Why would I ever want to move back to Pekin?" Dick, always the skeptic, loves to travel to new and different places and frequently asks my brother to join him. Bill said he has been fortunate to see the world with Dick, otherwise he never would have gone to some of the places, like Thailand or Nicaragua. The answer to Dick's question, of course, came two years later.

It took awhile for me to get grounded in Pekin. That always happens when I move to a new location. In other words, my charkas[1] need to reconnect to the earth so I can feel safe.

Before I moved to Pekin, I talked to my former friend Doug and told him I'd pay rent to live with him. Interestingly, he ended up in Pekin five years earlier by "accident." Of course there are no accidents, only coincidences. I had visited my brother for Thanksgiving one year and invited Doug to

---

1   chakras

join us from where he was living near St. Louis. He hadn't been working for quite awhile, so my brother offered him work.

Since I was unable to find work in Pekin, I applied at Tazewell County School District to be a substitute teacher. During that time and because I couldn't find a job, I applied for unemployment benefits from Reno. Reno delayed, put me off, and eventually, over a year later, denied my application.

I had my second seizure over ten months later.

Over the next year and a half, I experienced several seizures. One of them happened in the middle of the night, and I awoke not knowing exactly where I was. Then, I had a seizure for which I was mostly conscious. My right side became weaker as I fell backwards and could not stand up. I found myself lifting my right arm with my left hand and placing it in my lap. Within about ten minutes, I had all my movement back.

One would think that I'd be more concerned about these episodes/seizures. However, they were so far apart in time, I never gave them much consideration.

"Whatever you ask for in prayer with faith, you will receive."

Matthew 21:22

CHAPTER 4

DISCOVERY

On September 29, 2011, I had a seizure that scared me. I vaguely remember hanging up my towel in the bathroom. What seemed like moments later, I awoke on my couch. Apparently I walked or crawled from the bathroom to the living room where I found myself sitting on my couch. I then regained consciousness. Of course, *I do not remember any of this!*

After the September 29th episode, I finally decided to see a doctor. I told the doctor about my seizures and black outs. Prior to this, it crossed my mind that I must certainly have epilepsy, and I fully expected that to be the diagnosis. I even allowed myself to believe it and researched epilepsy drugs. That was a big step for me as I considered being on epilepsy drugs. I normally do not take any prescription drugs nor do I wish to. I had become very "holistic" in the last twenty years and even healed myself of breast cancer[2].

All of this reminded me of an experience with Debbie's husband, Jim. Debbie was my best friend from my college days. We were Resident Advisors in the all-girl's dorm one year. After she graduated from our college, she attended the University of Southern California where she earned her degree in Library Science after which she landed an interview in Ashland, Oregon with Southern Oregon College. I remember driving there with Debbie and Jim because Ashland is famous for its Shakespeare Festival. Debbie and I lost touch in the mid-1990's, but then she contacted me early in 2011. She said, "I don't want to lose touch with you again." Little did I know, the timing was perfect.

Jim, Debbie's husband, had three cancerous brain tumors right after they moved to Ashland. It was not a positive experience. When I told Debbie about my black outs, she was concerned and thought I may have a brain tumor. I, of course, simply dismissed it because I didn't want to consider that possibility. Yet, it struck me as very odd that she would

---

2   breast cancer

say something like that. I never considered a brain tumor. No way. It's impossible that I had a brain tumor! Yet, I was about to discover the impossible.

My doctor ordered several tests which included blood tests, an electroencephalogram (EEG) and a Magnetic Resonance Imaging Scan (MRI).

Because of the seizures, I asked my neighbor to drive me to the tests. First was the EEG, then the MRI. The MRI was in Morton where they offer a variety of videos and music. I was told the noise from the MRI was very, very loud which was news to me because I never had one before.

While at the MRI clinic, I asked if I would find out anything before I left. The tech wasn't sure. Yet in the end, I was asked to call a doctor for the results. I was surprised.

"You said you wanted to know something," the tech said.

"Yes." Yet I was scared of what I'd hear. I was very nervous and almost couldn't get dressed.

With the doctor on the phone, I was told rather matter-of-factly, **"You have a brain tumor and it needs to come out."**

What!!!!

My world stopped. Tears started. I was in shock.

I strained to hear every word the doctor told me on the phone. He gave me details on how to contact my regular physician, and have that information faxed to a neurologist for follow up. The doctor then asked if I could leave my car in Morton and take a cab home. That indicated to me that it was *very* serious.

I felt like crying, yet knew this wasn't the time or place. I'd been referred to a neurologist. How incredible is that? A neurologist! I was still trying to digest that information. It was like "before" knowing about the tumor, and "after" knowing about it. I never expected to hear the words, "you have a brain tumor."

In that moment, I knew I couldn't rely on any natural or holistic method. Not for this anyway. I'd written a book entitled *Natural Solutions, Women's Health Conditions*[3]. It is about balancing hormones through alternative choices. I did lots of research before writing that book. I knew alternatives were out of the question. Afterall, I was dealing with a brain tumor. I didn't know how to deal with it. I'd never had a brain tumor or brain surgery before.

I was referred to Illinois Nuerological Institute (INI) by my personal physician. He said that was the group they used.

My records were faxed to INI on Thursday, and by the following Monday I started to receive calls. I was scheduled to meet with Dr. Andrew Tsung on Tuesday at noon, and surgery was scheduled for that Thursday. This was moving very quickly. The

---

3   my book

advantage is there was no time to worry, although I didn't sleep for that entire week.

I decided to wait before calling my brother, Bill, who had recently left for Florida with his wife Connie. I was in shock and needed extra time to integrate the significance of all this. By late in the afternoon I was ready to call Bill. Connie was due to fly back that Thursday but without Bill. As it turned out, Bill flew back with Connie.

"Hi Bill."

"What's going on?"

"I'm afraid I have some news and it's not very good."

"What is it?" he asked calmly. He is rarely shaken by anything.

"I have a brain tumor."

"What?"

"I have a brain tumor and it has to come out." I don't know why I felt so odd saying these words to him, but I did. I didn't want him to go out of his way or fly back on my account.

He remained cool and calm though I could tell he was concerned. He said something to Connie under his breath which I interpreted as serious.

"I will keep you informed of everything as I find out more information." I said.

"Okay. We'll be waiting to hear."

I was anxious. I kept thinking about Steve Jobs who was in the news lately and had recently passed away. Early on, he could have taken a different road other than the alternative one that he chose. He had been diagnosed with pancreatic cancer and chose to do alternatives for the next nine months. The news media announced he could have taken a surgical approach which would have insured his survival to this day. I don't know if that's all true, but even if this is all hearsay, I listened to it anyway and pondered his outcome. I also thought about mine and came to the conclusion there were no "natural" or "alternative" choices available to me, at least not at this time.

My friend, Pat, drove me to the one-story brick building with INI letters on the side. I asked her to join me in the consultation. She did and stayed the entire time, taking notes, asking questions, and helping me to understand the ins and outs of brain surgery. I needed as much information as possible about this brain surgery stuff. My only question was whether I'd need a catheter. The answer was "yes," but it would be put in after I was already unconscious. That's funny that I would only think about that.

My appointment with Dr. Andrew Tsung went well. He is a little man, smaller than me, with very delicate hands. He's about thirty-five years old and yet looks much younger. I felt totally confident in his presence.

Dr. Tsung asked if I'd seen the tumor.

"No," I responded.

He took me into a room where he showed me an image on a computer. I was surprised to see it on the screen. It was about three by two inches by one-half inch! Big for a brain tumor. How could something like this grow in my head and I not know anything about it?

He said it was a meningioma (see Chapter 12) which is a fairly common type of tumor. (Meningiomas are generally benign and found most often in women from ages thirty to seventy). There are many other tumors, yet this is the one I have. The tumor names were all greek (or rather latin) to me. He said that when autopsied about ten to twenty percent of people have little meningiomas in their brain about the size of a finger tip but they do not grow. Mine had grown very large over twenty years or more. He did not know what caused it and neither did I. He was concerned about the size.

The cause of the meningioma could possibly be brain trauma. Let's see, do I remember any brain traumas? Was it when I fell down the stairs a few years ago. Probably not, because it wouldn't have had time to grow that big. Did I have headaches? No. Well sometimes, but generally no. It is a mystery.

I confidently believe the meditation I'd been doing for over twenty years made a significant difference. I was totally unaware of it until I had my first seizure in 2009. Even at that point, I did not know it was a brain tumor.

Dr. Tsung said it would take six to twelve hours to remove the tumor. I was surprised by this. Then he said I would be on anticonvulsants and steroids for about one month. That was the good news because I'd rather not be on any medications at all.

He went on to explain strokes, whether the tumor was benign or cancerous, that it was a very bloody surgery and they'd have at least six units of blood on hand. He didn't know if he'd get one-hundred percent of the tumor or not. He explained that I might have had some small hemorrhages when I had my seizures. At that point, I told him I'd been out for about forty-five minutes with the last seizure, and he was *very* concerned to say the least.

I was open for the tumor to be removed surgically, and I was totally amazed by the lightening speed with which it all occurred. One week I'm diagnosed with a tumor, and the next, I'm having surgery.

I was filled with doubt and fear if I'd come out of the surgery the same as I was or whether I'd be different or even possibly die. I did not know.

"Some changes look negative on the surface but you will soon realize that space is being created in your life for something new to emerge."

Eckhart Tolle, The Power of Now

CHAPTER 5

I TELL EVERYONE

Telling everyone about my tumor was a cathartic experience because I needed to speak up for myself and ask for help. I had been hiding behind my fear and denial for too long, and this brought it all into the light. I was challenged to tell people what was happening to me because I was almost embarrassed by the tumor and what I interpreted as a weakness and my lack of independence. This was a big step towards the healing of my soul. Unbelieveably to me, people stepped up to help in many ways. That is the benefit of living in a small town!

I informed Kathy, the choir director, that I'd not be coming to choir practice for awhile because I had a brain tumor. I can't remember if I told her by phone or in person. I could never get used to saying that. It felt strange and unusual. I'd never had a brain tumor before and never expected to have one. Yet I had one and felt uncomfortable with so much attention. It was hard for me to ask for help especially from people I hardly knew. (I had only been in the choir for about six months and we were off for three of those during the summer). This was now October. Kathy was a great help in communicating my situation to the choir, asking for prayers, and she informed many other people as well. I'm truly grateful for all the prayers and blessings of the choir that came my way. It restored my faith in people and in God.

My friend Pat was an earth angel. She accompanied me to my doctor appointments and is my dear friend. This experience has brought my friends together in ways that are surprising. Yet, isn't that what's supposed to happen; bringing people together through shared joy and tragedy.

I told Doug, my former boyfriend, about the tumor. He laughed and said "Maybe that's a good thing." Though I was irritated by his response, I realized later perhaps it *was* a good thing.

At Pekin Library I returned books. Pat and I informed them I had a brain tumor and would be having surgery that week. One of the ladies offered to bring a bag of books to my home on the first Tuesday of the month as long as I needed them. In one way I was surprised by this, and in another way, I wasn't. Everyone was extremely helpful and this was just another way it showed.

I told a couple people where I lived about the tumor. However, I requested that it not be common knowledge because I didn't want the attention.

Of course, I told my brother, Bill. Though he didn't tell me at the time, he was planning to fly back from Florida with his wife, Connie.

I had fears of dieing or not coming out of the anesthesia. I even made a list of contacts to be informed in case of my demise. I sent it to my brother as well as directions for my funeral. I had a DNR (Do Not Resuscitate) form that I gave to the hospital when I checked in. Yet, that all turned out not to be essential because, in retrospect, I had no earthly reason to be concerned. Though, at the time I was very worried. Fear means "False Evidence Appearing Real." I now know it was a false fear. It all seems very amusing now, but it wasn't at the time.

"Extreme remedies are very appropriate for extreme diseases."

Hippocrates

CHAPTER 6

SURGERY DAY

Today is the day of my surgery; my *brain surgery*. How surreal is that? It began quite early. Pat picked me up at five o'clock in the morning, and we arrived at OSF Hospital around five thirty. We checked in, and a nurse guided us to a small end space where lots of people were being prepped for surgery.

I was afraid. However, I couldn't turn back at this point. I had to "bite the bullet" and follow through. Would I be normal? Would I be incapacitated? Would I be a vegetable? Though I feared the outcome, I was calm and had a deeper sense of peace.

Until this moment, I had been very attracted to holistic and natural forms of healing, such as nutrition, herbs, meditation, aromatherapy, angels and much, much more. I'd self-published a book entitled "*Natural Solutions, Women's Health Conditions*" which talks about natural hormones and my journey to find wholeness and balance through menopause. As I was defining it for myself, I was explaining it to other women. Dr. Tsung had mentioned that hormones could be involved with the tumor. However, this was entirely different and knew I couldn't rely on natural methods. Perhaps, someone else could, but not me.

I followed the nurse's directions. She explained everything in great detail especially about the blue pen marks she made on my head. She suggested I keep the pen in my pocket saying, "Now, if the doctor asks to use this, you keep it." I smiled.

Then, I was taken for another MRI. At OSF, they were a little more rustic than the one in Morton. Earplugs, cloth over my eyes. Very high tech...hahaha! This particular MRI was designated as a Number Two, and it apparently shows more detail which Dr. Tsung would use during surgery. Fortunately, it only took about fifteen minutes.

As I was taken back to my little cubby hole, there sat a gentleman I recognized from two years ago when my niece died in a car accident. I didn't remember his name, so I asked him.

"Bob." He came from my brother's Monday morning prayer group.

"Good to see you," I said.

"How are *you?*" he asked.

"Doing pretty well."

The nurse was sitting right next to me working on her computer, apparently getting everything up-to-date and current for Dr. Tsung. I didn't know if we would interrupt her, so I asked, "Can we pray while Bob is here?"

We sat in a circle of four including the nurse, which surprised me, and Bob said a prayer while we all held hands.

"Dear Father, we ask that this procedure goes well for Ann and she come out from this completely healed. We want to thank You, Lord, for everything and know that this is divinely guided in your hands. Please guide the hands of all the people involved, the surgeons, nurses, and we pray for a positive outcome. We pray this in Jesus name, Amen." I loved the words and then as quickly as he arrived, he was gone.

Pat took all my clothes and walked me to where she left my side in the corridor. I held on to some lip gloss which was in my upper right pocket. That was my security. I was wheeled to the surgery room which brought up memories of having my tonsils removed when I was only five years old. As the doors to the surgery room opened, I was struck by all the technology around me...the people and machines.

I was introduced to techs with masks over their faces as I was wheeled over to an operating table where I was slid from the gurney to the table. This is all I remember because at that moment, I blacked out just like the nurse had told me.

SAME DAY...AFTER SURGERY

Wow! Amazing! Where was I? What happened?

I was groggy as I began to regain consciousness. I heard through the dense fog of my mind the surgery was under three hours. That was a surprise because both I and Dr. Tsung expected it to last at least six to twelve hours. At this point, I was on a gurney next to a nurse's station.

The nurse was talking on the phone attempting to find a place for me. Rooms were apparently at a premium. I was eventually moved to the ICU. It had a beautiful view of the downtown skyline. I could've looked at the lights all night.

I heard the nurses ask each other if they could bring in my "Significant Other."

"Yes," I whispered and nodded.

I heard this through my fogged mind with my eyes closed. I wondered who the "Significant Other" was because my brother wasn't back from Florida yet. Maybe it was Pat. But in came Lewie, my nephew! He brought little footies and headbands for me. He didn't know that my head wasn't shaved. It was only shaved along the incision line. Yet, that was very thoughtful of him.

He had poked his head in earlier and didn't recognize me because my face was bloated. He went to the nurses station to ask if it was really me. They assured him it was. He had stayed around all that day telling me it was actually "fun" to be doing something and not be bored at home. He had shoulder surgery not too long ago and is limited to what he can do. He finally felt useful. Thanks Lewie.

Throughout the day, Lewie kept my brother, Bill, informed by phone. Lewie also met with Dr. Tsung who gave him the details of the surgery. One of the reasons the surgery went so quickly was the tumor was not attached to any main arteries, and I only needed two units of blood.

Lewie commented that Dr. Tsung was a "little" man, and Lewie isn't that big himself.

The nursing staff was great, and communicated with me to take vitals. They checked my awareness by asking questions.

"Where are you?"

"Hospital" I answered.

"Why are you here?"

"Brain tumor."

"What year is it?" I had a problem with this one, but managed to answer," 2011."

Of course, one night I answered in a fog, "1968." They asked what happened that year and I said my Dad died. Afterall, what do they expect being awakened from a deep sleep in the middle of the night?

"Who is the President?"

"Obama." I answered.

I would be asked these questions several times during the day and night, so they would know if my brain was working and also to check my awareness. It was a little difficult on my part to come up with the answers when they first asked. Yet, I can understand why they ask so frequently because events can change so quickly and without warning especially with the brain.

Watching the clock that night, time moved very slowly. It was 2:00 a.m., then 2:10 a.m, then 2:20 a.m. Time really dragged, as I went in and out of consciousness. Lights were on in the room. People were bustling around. This is not a good way to get a restful night's sleep!

The nursing staff took vitals about every three to four hours. I "heard" my blood sugar was 190, then 185. My blood sugar fluctuated so much that I was given a shot of insulin. I had two intravenous units in my arms where I was receiving antibiotics and other medications, plus an oxygen delivery system. Plus I had a catheter that I was grateful for because I didn't have the energy to get up.

All in all from what I could tell, the surgery went very well and I had all my faculties back.

"Your life is what your thoughts make it."

Marcus Aurelius

CHAPTER 7

DAY AFTER SURGERY

The day after surgery, I found myself in the intensive care unit (ICU). My face was swollen and puffy. My eyes swelled up even more, and I couldn't see very well. I avoided looking in the mirror, yet when I did, I was shocked. My face had no definition. It was puffy and round. I didn't recognize myself! No wonder Lewie couldn't recognize me right after surgery! I made a note to get ice for my face. I used many techniques to reduce the swelling and relieve the pressure. My face was hot, and it felt so good to hold my cool hands over my face.

I was grateful that I had most of my hair. Dr. Tsung had only shaved the area where he made the incision. It was quite a large incision going from one ear to the other over the top of my head.

When the nurse brought my medications, I took them the first day. The next day I objected to the amount. Too many. They originally wanted me to take 1000 milligrams two times a day of the anti-convulsant. I only agreed to take 500 milligrams twice a day, and even objected to that. After all, I hadn't taken any medications up to that point.

I took steroids in the amount of 1000 milligrams four times a day. Again, I felt that was too much, so I began to cut it back. However, one of the doctors said it released the swelling in the brain so I agreed to take it. However, I knew I'd only be on these for one short month.

On Friday, I got the last intravenous injection of antibiotics. I was on steroids, anti-convulsants, plus stool softeners which don't do anything for me, and I said so. The pain medication more than "stops" me up.

What a day! I was "out" for most of it; unconscious then conscious. Hearing everyone, seeing everything, I knew I was feeling better and the surgery was a success. Yeah! I wondered when my brother and Connie would show up. They didn't arrive back in town until late the night before as they were traveling back from Florida.

Bill and Connie arrived mid-morning. Bill walked in first, then Connie. I hugged both of them. Because I was stuck in the hospital without anything to do, they offered to get a book to keep me entertained. The book was delivered later in the day. It arrived through the hospital mail system. It was entitled *"The Help"* by Kathryn Stockett. Bill wrote inside the cover "Get Well, Love, Bill + Connie." The book was about Jackson, Mississippi in the sixty's, and actually, I graduated from high school in Little Rock, Arkansas during that time. So it brought back many memories of how much I disliked living in the South.

Later in the day, Pat showed up. She held my toes to keep them warm. It felt so good; I asked her to massage my hands and back. I guided her, and she did a terrific job.

I continued to help myself heal using the following techniques. I used holistic tools consistently for several years *before* the surgery, and now I also used them *after* surgery.

Sword Fingers[4] is a Qigong (*"Spring Forest Qigong, Level 2 for Healing,"* Master Chunyi Lin, 2001) technique where I use the first two fingers of one hand to break up negative or dark energy by moving them

---

4   Sword Fingers

back and forth over the spot that needs healing. I used that technique over my head where the incision had been made. I found myself visualizing that I was pulling dark strings out of my head along that line. I used the visualization to pull out negative energy. To help myself be more precise, I would close my eyes to use my imagination. I visualized strings coming out of my head where the staples were. After I pulled out the dark energy, I threw it away by taking clumps and tossing it aside. Then, I gently put positive energy back. I did that by holding my palm with closed fingers and gently cupping back positive energy in the same area. This felt very wonderful, and I did it frequently.

Then I used a ***mantra meditation practice***[5]. I repeated *Sa Ta Na Ma* over and over. This helped me feel calmer. In fact, it felt very relaxing and peaceful while doing it. Following is the technical explanation of the mantra as stated in "*Meditation as Medicine, Activate the Power of Your Natural Healing Force.*[6]" (*Page 122*).

"*This mantra which is used in the important Kirtan Kriya, is called the Panch Shabd, or Primal Sound Mantra because it consists of five primal sounds. S, T, N, M and ah. The literal meaning is as follows: Sa means birth (or*

5   Mantra Meditation
6   Meditation as Medicine

infinity); Ta means life; Na means death; and Ma means rebirth.

The physical benefits of the mantra are:

- *Sa evokes a sense of emotion and expansiveness.*
- *Ta creates a feeling of transformation and strength.*
- *Na stimulates a feeling of universal love.*
- *Ma evokes a quality of communicativeness.*

(Another description of these three modes of speech is that they are, respectively, the voice of the body, the mind and the spirit.)"

This technique was very appropriate as it takes one from birth to death and then rebirth.

Throughout the day, I also used a "tapping" technique known as EFT[7] *(Emotional Freedom Technique)* the tapping technique, developed by Gary Craig. I tapped from the top of my eyebrows, down seven points on my face (side of eye, under eye, under nose, under chin, the clavicle point, under my arm and then back to the top of my head which is number eight.) I tapped *very* gently repeating words to the effect "Even though I had this brain tumor, it is now gone and I deeply and completely love and accept myself." I practiced this several times during the day. These are "tried and true" techniques and can be found easily on the internet.

---

7   EFT

I practiced these techniques several times throughout the day and I know they helped me relax and, most importantly, heal more quickly.

Later that day, I was moved to another room. That room was also very nice. It had a view plus it was a room by myself. I had the catheter removed as well as one of the intravenous tubes and the oxygen. I was left with one intravenous line and a blood pressure cuff. Of course, when I got up to go to the bathroom, buzzers went off and a nurse rushed in. They were afraid I would fall, even though I never did. Yet, I can understand their concern.

"Patterning your life around other's opinions is nothing more than slavery."

Lawana Blackwell

CHAPTER 8

DINNER WITH DOUG

Shortly after I got home from my surgery, I attended a dinner with Doug, my former boyfriend and recent roommate. I felt tired this day but got dressed anyway.

The restaurant was filled with many of Doug's friends. After the dinner, Steve took over as Master of Ceremonies. Steve is the minister who came to the hospital to meet with me after my surgery and called Doug's "Prayer Chain." He offered prayers for everyone at the dinner and then began to present awards. Roses were passed around as were little bird houses called "Birdhouses of Prayer." Each one of these was handcrafted by Steve.

Then, Steve brought out a hundred year old Bible. He created a story from the mementos he found in the Bible, i.e. a piece of cloth, two calling cards and a newspaper notice.

Steve speculated that the piece of cloth could have been from a wedding dress or a baptismal gown. The two cards could have been "calling cards" from male pursuers or perhaps even rivals for the lady. The newspaper notice could have been from some kind of special event. Who knows? Perhaps we never will. However, this experience sparked my imagination enough to write this book.

Before it was over, people were asking me about my brain surgery. I can truly say that I feel lighter, more open, more transformed especially by the love and genuine concern of people around me, by all the prayers I received and by life in general.

Additionally, I learned to slow down and savor special moments like these. It's as though the pressure has been lifted off my head. I'm calmer, more focused, and happier over all.

Perhaps this is why I feel so free from all fears. I don't try so hard to please others. In fact, I don't try to do anything except be myself.

"It takes a long time to become young."

Picasso

CHAPTER 9

HELEN VISITS

One evening after I had returned home, Helen showed up at my door. Kathy, the choir director, suggested she stop by and say hello to me. One simply does not ignore a "suggestion" from Kathy as Helen said. Interestingly, Helen was also my mother's name, and she did remind me very much of my dear mother.

I asked her to tell me about herself. I had heard her name before. In fact, Kathy had asked me if I knew her, but unfortunately, I didn't.

Helen sat on the couch, and we talked and talked. She reminded me so much of my mother. How time flies. First it's third grade, when I assisted in crowning the May Queen (Mother Mary) and then it's 2011 and I'm sixty-three years old! We talked about many of the kids in my early school classes at St. Joseph Catholic School.

Helen said she remembered my brother, Bill. I didn't realize she knew him. "He's memorable," said I. My brother tended to be a rabble-rouser. He was a let's-make-trouble-just-for-the-heck-of-it kind of a kid, so to speak. Yet he always came out spotless in the end.

Then Helen said the strangest thing. She said my dad used to talk about the "big open skies of Madison (Wisconsin)."

In that moment, it was very clear to me that **MY DAD HAD DREAMS!** What a special revelation. It struck me like a bolt of lightening. I think about what they might have been. My Dad's dreams. My Dad had dreams! My Dad had dreams. Of course, he did. We all do.

I continually ask myself, "What were his dreams?" I see my dad looking out the window in Madison looking at the pristine snow. He'd get upset whenever a deer or dog walked across it leaving its footprints behind. Was he wondering, thinking, dreaming, contemplating? He'd sit at the kitchen table with both feet flat on the floor, holding a cigarette in both hands, gazing off in the distance at something not there. Was he dreaming then? Perhaps dreaming of something more wonderful than what he had in the moment.

I've had many issues to work out with my father over the years. Unfortunately, I have not spent too much time considering how he was feeling. Now that I heard it from someone other than my mother, I am very aware that my Dad had dreams, and I truly wonder what they were.

"Realize deeply that the present moment is all you have. Make the NOW the primary focus of your life."

Eckhart Tolle, The Power of Now: A Guide to Spiritual Enlightenment

CHAPTER 10

RECUPERATION

Okay. So, I've been recuperating for twenty days now. I am better, and yet worse. My head is swollen and I seem to be oozing liquid from my brain. Makes me very tired. Yet I have all my faculties for which I am truly grateful. Seeing, breathing, hearing, comprehending, yet I'm not highly motivated. Being tired, I lack energy to work or get things done. Mostly I want to sit and relax. This surgery apparently has been a very big deal from which it will take awhile to recover. Not knowing that from the beginning is probably better.

One week after the surgery I had the staples removed from my scalp. I was fearful that it would hurt, but the nurse promised it wouldn't. It didn't hurt one bit.

However I do pray and think about things. Things simply don't seem as important as they did before. I am clear-headed, yet removed to a certain degree. I feel like I'm not fully back in my body.

It's kind of interesting that I'm not farther along. I've learned to slow down, to relax, to let things go, to just sit and not have too much movement. Though I've meditated for many years, it's important to learn these things again. Time is allowed to just be. Yes, be in the moment as Eckhart Tolle expresses in *The Power of Now*[8]. This is what I am learning to do. I pray I continue to have these perceptions.

ONE MONTH INTO RECUPERATION

One month after my surgery, I had an appointment with the Physician Assistant. Once again, Pat went with me to the appointment.

I asked if Dr. Tsung had been able to get one hundred percent of the tumor. She replied, "yes." Then she told me the labs came back, and it was designated as a Meningioma Grade II which is considered benign. Hurray! All is well.

---

8   Power of Now

She also informed me that the tumor was not attached to any major arteries. However, it was attached to my skull. So the skull had to be "scraped" to get the tumor off.

I asked for a copy of a picture of the tumor and was informed she would try to find one. Later she told me there wasn't one available; that it was from someone else's surgery.

TWO MONTHS INTO RECUPERATION

Again, I met with Dr. Tsung's Assistant. She informed me that she was not able to locate a copy of the picture. However, she did give me a copy of the labs. I couldn't really understand them however.

I had an MRI about two weeks earlier. I asked what the results of the MRI were. She said that Dr. Tsung had talked with Dr. McGee who is a radiologist, and she wanted me to consider a couple radiation treatments. This was to prevent the tumor from growing back. Of course, I did not want to do this, but agreed to talk to Dr. McGee. So, I made an appointment to see him.

A couple weeks later I met with Dr. McGee. He was reading information from a computer screen where Federal Government Guidelines are posted. He told me a Meningioma Grade III would require some radiation, but a Meningioma Grade I or II could not be agreed upon by the panel. So I did not agree to radiation, nor did he suggest it. Now, I feel I am home free. I do need to have an MRI in another six months and another one a year after that. Fortunately, I look at the NOW as the most important and only time to be alive, and I do appreciate life in the moment.

SIX MONTHS INTO RECUPERATION

I had a seizure exactly six months into recuperation. Boy, was I surprised! Up until that time, I was driving, wasn't taking any medication, and hadn't had any seizures since having my brain surgery. In fact, I made a big mistake by walking up eight flights of stairs which triggered my seizure. After spending a night at the hospital and having an MRI, I went back on my medication and stopped driving.

Then, one month following that I had another seizure while I was at choir practice. I hadn't taken any medication that day and, in fact, commented to Pat that I was experimenting with not taking it. Of course, she told me all about what happened after I passed out. She said I was "out" for a good twenty minutes, and it took an additional ten minutes to get my bearings when I came back. People were talking to me but I couldn't answer them. In fact, I don't even remember what was said to me. I had no indication of the oncoming seizure, yet I do remember turning in a circle and following my eyes until I passed out. That didn't happen the last time. All the choir members were very concerned, even though they knew what had happened. I am very grateful to have been with my choir family as they knew exactly what to do and who to call. They called 911, and they called the pastor from the church to give me last rites. This experience let me know that I would be on my medication for the rest of my life. Though I'm somewhat disappointed, I will adjust, and I don't want to cause any harm to myself or others.

"To appeal to God is to appeal to the action of universal love."

Marianne Williamson, Illumanata

CHAPTER 11

10 STEPS TO FOLLOW IF YOU ARE DIAGNOSED WITH A BRAIN TUMOR

If you are diagnosed with a brain tumor, here are steps to follow to find out what you can do and what to expect:

1. PAY ATTENTION TO THE MESSAGES YOUR BODY GIVES YOU. Your body is very wise. It knows what's going on, and it's important

for you to learn to read the signs. DO NOT IGNORE any seizure or blackout.

2. DO NOT PANIC. Of course, this is easier said then done. However, if you can remain calm and focused, you will follow through with what you need to do. I was unconsciously guided to know what to do, and of course, I was prepared by my previous meditation and prayer work. Neale Donald Walsch says that "medical conditions are nothing to be afraid of when God is on your side." (Internet newsletter "*I Believe God Wants You to Know.*"). Of course, God is always on your side.

3. BE PREPARED TO MAKE CHANGES IN YOUR STATE OF BODY AND MIND. Please know it's important to "find" yourself. You do that by knowing who you are, what you want, and how you feel about yourself and others. Once again, pay attention to the emotions you feel in your body and mind.

4. GET ALL THE INFORMATION YOU CAN. This is very important. If you don't trust yourself to take good notes, then take a friend or family member with you to visit the neurologist. I did. I had many questions, which my friend asked, and I ended up with more information than I would have otherwise. This is key. You

can then refer back to what was said if you have questions after the surgery.

5. PREPARE YOURSELF FOR THE OUTCOME. This again, is easier said then done. Unfortunately, I had several sleepless nights prior to my surgery. Though I didn't expect anything but the "best" outcome, I was very nervous. I can't expect you to be any less worried than I was, but knowing this first is helpful. Remember, it's important to *believe* in a positive outcome.

6. SURROUND YOURSELF WITH POSITIVE, SUPPORTIVE PEOPLE. I had a wonderful support group with my family and church choir. They prayed for me and actually helped drive me around (it was suggested that I not drive because of my seizures which I was having without warning). This suggestion is one that continues *after* the surgery as well. Continuing with the positive interaction after surgery is extremely helpful not only with recovery, but with choosing a way to live.

7. BE AWARE THAT YOU WILL BE TRANSFORMED IN MANY WAYS. Expect to experience changes to your life, your personality, and your cognitive abilities once you have surgery. This can be an enlightening experience or a difficult one. For example, I am a

little more tired yet actually more patient than I've ever been before. Whatever happens, just know it was meant to be. It's a "soul" lesson of the most significant type.

8. FOLLOW UP CONDITIONS. I was very fortunate in that I did not have any follow up problems, i.e. cancer or treatments for it. In fact, I had the very "best" outcome and needed no radiation or chemotherapy. However, if you should need these treatments, be sure to discuss them with someone who can help you direct where the radiation should go or the chemo that is to be used. As a trained hypnotherapist, I know you can visualize those treatments being targeted to the problem areas. On the other hand, find someone in your area who is trained in hypnotherapy or alternative health. Personally, I chose not to do radiation even though it was suggested to prevent the tumor from growing back. The reason is because I employ and believe in alternative practices such as meditation, qi gong, yoga and prayer. In fact, I see my life as a spiritual journey that offers soul lessons along the way.

9. RECOVERY. Expect your recovery to last a couple months, perhaps more or perhaps less. In my case, I healed very quickly. That was partially because I was so healthy going into the

surgery. However, when I got home, I was extremely tired for a couple months. This is to be expected.

10. EXPECTATIONS.   Do not hold any expectations. However, expect anything and everything!

"Life isn't as serious as the mind makes it out to be."

Eckhart Tolle, The Power of Now, A Guide to Spiritual Enlightenment

CHAPTER 12

INFORMATION ABOUT MENINGIOMAS

A lot of information on brain tumors has been in the news lately. By far, the most common type of brain tumor is known as a meningioma. Meningiomas are generally benign. Mine was, and even though it was designated as a Meningioma Grade II, it did not require any chemotherapy or radiation.

A meningioma is a tumor that grows from the meninges, which is the membrane that surrounds the brain and spinal cord. In fact, when I was experiencing seizures, I was hoping I'd simply pass out and never wake up again, but obviously, that was not to be.

Meningiomas can grow fast or slow. A meningioma usually grows on the surface of the brain toward the front of the head. It can reach a rather large size, at which point it may cause symptoms. That is what mine did. It could have been growing for up to twenty or thirty years. I believe I knew it was there two years prior to my surgery because I experienced a seizure. I just didn't know that's what I experienced. I was fortunate that I did not have more than one tumor as several meningiomas can grow at one time. A meningioma is the most common type of brain tumor and occurs mostly in women between the ages of forty and seventy.

Diagnosis for a brain tumor is usually an MRI. My symptoms were seizures, and I never knew when they would happen. One time I was standing in my kitchen when I unexpectedly had a minor seizure. My right side went weak and I fell backwards on to the floor. I didn't pass out as I did the other times. I had to lift my right arm up on my lap. When I noticed feeling coming back, I could stand and started to use my right hand and arm again . Yet, I never experienced headaches, memory loss or unsteadiness, which are also symptoms.

The cause of meningiomas is often related to radiation or previous head injury, or even sometimes hormones or viruses. However, the hormones and virus cause is not substantiated at this time.

If you want more information, please check out various sites on the internet.

ENDNOTES

1. Chakras. There are seven charkas (some people believe there are more). These are vortexes of energy corresponding to various places in the body. The seven are: First, the root chakra or kundalini which relates to one's grounding is located at the base of the spine; Second, the sacral chakra which relates to creativity and sexual needs; Third, is the solar plexus chakra, which relates to your physical power and is located at the stomach area; Fourth, the heart chakra which relates to all kinds of love; Fifth, the throat chakra which relates to one's speech and expression; Sixth, the Third Eye is located in the center of the forehead and relates to clairvoyance; and the Seventh, which is the crown of the head is our connection to Spirit.

2. Breast Cancer. I used many techniques to heal this condition including herbs, vitamins, angels and especially visualization, prayer and belief. I was able to obtain a healing in less than two months. It has not returned.

3. *Natural Solutions, Women's Health Conditions,* Ann Wesso, Self-published, 2002.

4. *Spring Forest Qigong, Level 2 for Healing,* Video, Master Chunyi Lin, 2001, Sword Fingers.

5. *Mantra Meditation Practice* is where you focus on a mantra. A mantra can be a word, a phrase, a sound or sacred words. *Sa Ta Na Ma* are sacred words.

6. *Meditation as Medicine, Activate the Power of Your Natural Healing Force,* Dharma Singh Khalsa, M.D. and Cameron Smith, Fireside Edition, 2002.

7. *Emotional Freedom Technique* (EFT), Homestudy Course, Tapping Technique discovered and promoted by Gary Craig,

8. *The Power of Now,* Eckhart Tolle, 2004, New World Library and Namaste Publishing.

ABOUT THE AUTHOR

Ann currently lives in Pekin, Illinois with her 19 year old cat, Josephine.

Her own personal and recent experience with a brain tumor prompted the writing of this book. She did not know anything about brain tumors. Yet, she learned a great deal in a short amount of time.

She has always been interested in health and healing, and as such became a Holistic Health Practitioner in 1995 while living in San Diego, California. At that same time, she obtained a certification as a Clinical Hypnotherapist, a Nutritionist, a Meditation Teacher, a trainer for Nuero Linguistic Programming, and as a Certified Spiritual Counsel (otherwise known as an Angeltherapist). She also earned a Bachelor of Arts degree in English from California State University at Northridge. She was the first one in her family to receive an advanced degree.

She wrote an earlier book in 2002 entitled, *Natural Solutions, Women's Health Conditions.* During that time, Ann developed breast cancer. To combat the cancer, Ann used all natural and alternative remedies to heal herself including meditation and visualization to "imagine" the tumor gone. Interestingly, in her first hypnotherapy class, she met a man who stated he had rid himself of cancer the very same way. This impressed her immensely, and when her time came, she utilized similar techniques.

Ann was born in 1948 in Illinois and was adopted in October the same year by the parents who raised her. In 2008, she returned to her home town of Pekin, where she now lives. She joined the choir at the Catholic Church where the choir members prayed and supported her through her most recent experience. Years ago Ann moved to several different states, including Arkansas where she graduated from high school, then to California where she earned her Bachelor of Arts in English Literature, then from there she moved to San Diego where she lived for twenty years. From there she moved to Las Vegas and then Reno. It was there that she had her first seizure and then drove all the way back to Pekin. By choice, Ann's never married, however, she's had many interesting life experiences.

PRAYER TO ST. FRANCIS OF ASSISI

Lord, make me an instrument of your peace
Where there is hatred, let me sow love.
Where there is injury, pardon.
Where there is discord, peace.
Where there is doubt, faith.
Where there is error, truth.
Where there is despair, hope.
Where there is sadness, joy.
Where there is darkness, light.

O Divine Master, grant that I may not so much seek
To be consoled, as to console.
To be understood, as to understand.
To be loved, as to love.

For
It is in giving, that we receive.
It is in pardoning, that we are pardoned.
It is in dying to self, that we are born to eternal life.

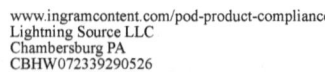